Najla MOUHLI

Mesotherapy Vs. Acupuncture in the treatment of cervicarthrosis

Najla MOUHLI

Mesotherapy Vs. Acupuncture in the treatment of cervicarthrosis

ScienciaScripts

Imprint

Any brand names and product names mentioned in this book are subject to trademark, brand or patent protection and are trademarks or registered trademarks of their respective holders. The use of brand names, product names, common names, trade names, product descriptions etc. even without a particular marking in this work is in no way to be construed to mean that such names may be regarded as unrestricted in respect of trademark and brand protection legislation and could thus be used by anyone.

Cover image: www.ingimage.com

This book is a translation from the original published under ISBN 978-620-6-71537-5.

Publisher:
Sciencia Scripts
is a trademark of
Dodo Books Indian Ocean Ltd. and OmniScriptum S.R.L publishing group

120 High Road, East Finchley, London, N2 9ED, United Kingdom
Str. Armeneasca 28/1, office 1, Chisinau MD-2012, Republic of Moldova, Europe
Printed at: see last page
ISBN: 978-620-8-09343-3

Contents

1 Introduction 2

2 Materials and methods 3

3 Results 6

4 Discussion 28

5 Conclusions 34

References 38

Appendices 42

1 Introduction

Chronic neck pain is a frequent reason for consultation, both in 1ere line facilities and in specialist consultations. In Western populations, they represent the 3eme most frequent musculoskeletal disorder [1]. They are a public health problem because of their disabling and recurrent nature, and their cost to the community. In fact, around 10% of patients with chronic neck pain suffer from physical incapacity and 5% from disability [2].

Treatment of this condition is multidisciplinary, involving the rheumatologist, the physical physician and sometimes the spinal surgeon. In addition to a wide range of drugs, the treatment includes appropriate rehabilitation [3]. In order to relieve patients' pain more effectively, the practitioner uses so-called complementary therapies, such as acupuncture or mesotherapy.

Acupuncture is a 4000-year-old form of traditional Chinese medicine [4]. Because of the diversity of its indications, its safety and its low cost, acupuncture is becoming more widely practised, and patient demand is growing. It is frequently used in rheumatology to relieve chronic pain, particularly neck pain [5]. Modern science has developed several theories to explain its efficacy, the most notable of which are the neuronal and neuro-endocrine theories. Its analgesic action is therefore thought to be due to the reinforcement of inhibitory influxes of type C sensory fibres [6,7], associated with the release of endogenous morphinomimetic peptides [8-10], thus explaining the effects induced near and far from the stimulated sites.

Mesotherapy is a relatively recent technique, introduced by Pistor in the 50s [11]. Its therapeutic concept is simple, consisting of bringing the site of therapy closer to the site of the disease. It acts at the level of the microcirculation, and the mesotherapeutic benefit is the result of the combination of a pharmacological product and the reflex effect of the puncture [3,12]. In fact, it combines analgesic and decontracting medications in a metameric segmental manner and in refractory cellulomyalgic painful areas [3]. Its value as an adjunctive therapy in the treatment of musculoskeletal pain, particularly chronic neck pain, is increasingly recognised [13].

The objectives of this work are :

-     To evaluate the clinical effectiveness of mesotherapy and acupuncture as complementary treatments for mechanical neck pain of degenerative origin.

-     To compare the efficacy of these two therapies in the short term.

2 Materials and methods

1] <u>Presentation of the study :</u>

This is a prospective study which took place between August 2015 and December of the same year. It involved 50 patients. The patients were divided into two groups.

The 1er group, comprising 25 patients, consulted the Acupuncture Department of the Mongi Slim Hospital in La Marsa. Tunis, Tunisia

The 2me group, comprising 25 patients, consulted the Physical Medicine and Functional Rehabilitation Department of the Institut Mohamed Kassab D'Orthopedie, Tunis, Tunisia.

2] <u>Inclusion, non-inclusion and exclusion criteria :</u>

Patients with common neck pain, of osteoarthritic origin, and with a response to the Visual Analogue Scale (VAS**)** for pain greater than or equal to 40/100 were included in the study.

Our study did not include patients with:

- Neck pain secondary to trauma.
- Neck pain associated with inflammatory rheumatism.
- Cervicalgia of infectious or tumoral origin, known as symptomatic cervicalgia.
- Cervicobrachial neuralgia.
- A sign of medullary distress or vertebral artery damage.
- A general illness affecting the functions of hemostasis or the use of anticoagulants

Patients who did not complete the entire treatment protocol were excluded from the study.

3] <u>The study protocol :</u>

The study protocol included :

a. <u>The V^{re} consultation:</u>

This pre-consultation enabled us to :

- Check inclusion and non-inclusion criteria.
- Obtaining informed oral consent from patients.
- Fill in the questionnaire (Appendix 1). In addition to the epidemiological data, the questionnaire asks patients to describe their neck pain (intensity assessed by the Visual Analogue Scale VAS, duration of evolution, notion of irradiation, associated signs, etc.), as well as the detailed physical examination of the cervical spine (limitation of mobility, postural abnormalities, etc.).

b. <u>The therapeutic protocol :</u>

The patients included in the study were divided into two groups:

- The 1er group: patients who consulted the acupuncture department of the CHU Mongi Slim in La Marsa, received a prescription for 10 sessions at a rate of 3 sessions per week. This prescription may or may not have been combined with conventional medical treatment (medication, rehabilitation, wearing a knee brace, etc.). The acupuncture treatment involved a combination of points, on average 8 to 10 points (Appendix 2):

- Puncture of local points (VB20, VB21, V11, DM14, PE21 cervical...)
- Standard distal puncture points for neck pain
- Puncture of Ashi points (local pain points)
- Puncturing the points according to the location of the pain (shoulder, scapula, upper limb)
- Applying electrical stimulation to the puncture needles. The electrical stimulation, with a frequency of 2 Hz, is applied to an average of 3 or 4 needles. The electro-acupuncture session lasted on average

of 20 minutes.

- Occasional cupping with or without scarification.
- The 2eme group: patients who consulted the Physical Medicine and Functional Rehabilitation department of the Mohamed Kassab Orthopaedic Institute were prescribed 3 mesotherapy sessions at a rate of one session per week. This prescription may or may not have been combined with conventional medical treatment (medication, rehabilitation, wearing a neck brace, etc.). The mesotherapeutic treatment consisted of a combination of 2 techniques: a series of deep intra-dermal injections of a mixture of : Lidocaine, thiocolchicoside and ketoprofen using a 13 mm needle, and superficial intradermal injections using a mixture of Lidocaine and thiocolchicoside using a 4 mm needle.

c. **A follow-up to Involution :**

A detailed clinical evaluation was carried out for the 1er group after the 3eme (A3) and 6eme (A6) acupuncture sessions, as well as at the end of the treatment. The second group had an assessment after each mesotherapy session (M1 and M2), which took place just before the next session. The last evaluation was carried out one week after the end of treatment. In addition to the objective clinical assessment, the patient was asked to report whether there had been any improvement (VAS), this being a subjective criterion.

A favourable response to treatment was established when, on re-evaluation of the pain, there was a 30% reduction in the VAS value compared with the initial value and/or an improvement in the amplitudes of the cervical spine with a reduction in the chin-sternum distances on flexion and extension, chin-acromion on right and left rotations and tragus of the ear-acromion on right and left lateral tilts, thus signifying greater flexibility of the neck. Another objective criterion for a favourable outcome was the improvement in any postural disorder, as assessed by the distances between the spinous processes of C3 and C7 and the plumb line (or wall). A value greater than 6.5 cm for C3-wall indicates anteprojection of the cervical spine, and a value greater than 4.5 cm for C7-wall indicates dorsal hypercyphosis, often associated with neck pain [14].

4] <u>Statistical analysis of data:</u>

Data was entered and analysed using SPSS® 17.01 (Statistical Package for Social Sciences, SPSS Inc, Chicago, Illinois). Graphs were produced using Excel® 12.0 (Microsoft Office 2007, Microsoft Corporation, Washington).

Descriptive and analytical studies were carried out.

a. <u>Descriptive study</u> :

We calculated simple frequencies and relative frequencies (percentages) for the qualitative variables. And means, standard deviations and extreme values were determined for the quantitative variables.

b. <u>Analytical study:</u>

- Comparison of percentages: The comparison of percentages on independent series was carried out using Person's chi-square test, and in the event of non-validity of this test, by Fisher's two-tailed exact test.

- Quantitative variables were compared between groups using the ANOVA test.

- In all statistical tests, the statistical significance level (p) was set at 0.05.

5] <u>Bibliographic research :</u>

A systematic review of the literature was also carried out. We selected English- and French-language articles published between 1976 and 2016 by consulting the Medline and Google Scholar databases. The keywords used alone or in combination were as follows: Acupuncture, Mesotherapy, mesotherapie, cervicalgies chroniques, chronic neck pain.

MATERIALS AND METHODS

We have also consulted the results of Tunisian work, which is mainly in the form of master's or CEC dissertations, as well as oral or poster communications.

6] <u>Ethical considerations :</u>

Informed consent was obtained orally from patients in both groups before the start of the therapeutic protocol.

We also declare that we have no conflicts of interest in relation to this study.

3 Results

1] **Descriptive study :**

a. **Overall description of the workforce:**

The total number of patients was 50, with an average age of 56.2 ±13.7 years, and extremes of 20 and 82 years. The majority of patients were between 50 and 70 years of age (Figure 1). There were 36 women and 14 men. Our patients had been suffering from neck pain for a mean of 6.1 years [min: 1 month, max: 25 years].

Breakdown of workforce by age

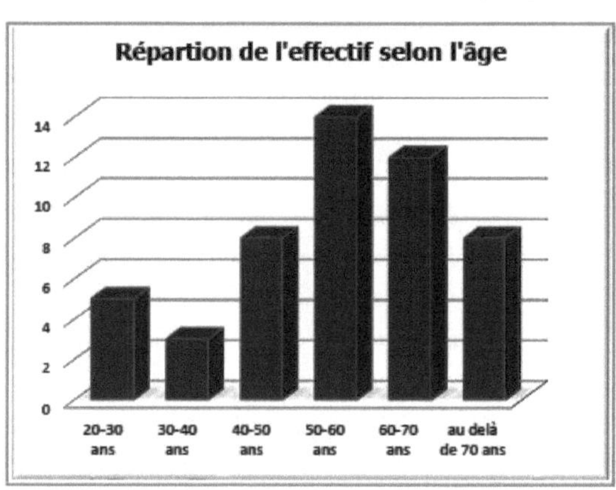

Figure 1: Breakdown of workforce by age

b. **Description of the 1ᵉʳ group (Acupuncture group):**

i. Demographic data :

The 1ᵉʳ group comprised 25 patients; 17 women and 8 men. Their average age was 57.5 ± 13.7 years [min: 20, max: 80 years]. Eight of them were manual workers, six had administrative jobs and the rest were either unemployed or retired.

ii. Description of symptoms and treatments received:

Neck pain had been evolving for a mean of 7.1 ± 6.7 years [min: 1 month, max: 25 years]. Pain radiated to the upper limb(s) in 64% of cases. In about 1/3 of cases, the radiations were poorly systematised (Figure 2). Neck pain was associated with tingling in the hands (52%), headache (40%), vertigo (48%) and tinnitus (28%).

Distribution of cervicalgia irradiation territories

in the 1st group

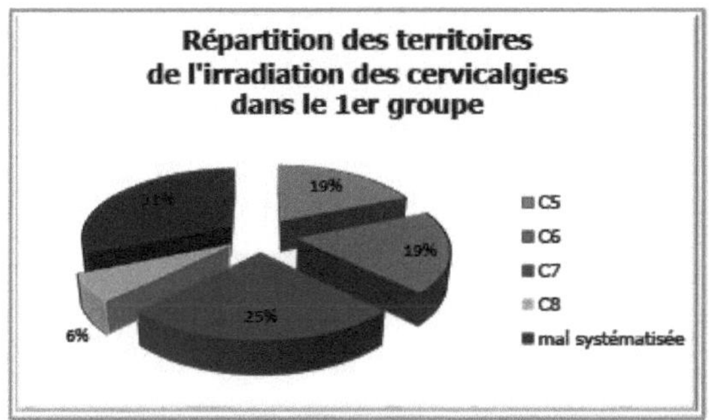

Figure 2: *Distribution of cervicalgia irradiation territories in the 1ᵉʳ group*

80% of patients in the group had received medical treatment in the last month, and 64% had benefited from rehabilitation in the last 6 months. The most commonly prescribed drugs were analgesics as required (80%), non-steroidal anti-inflammatory drugs (NSAIDs) (32%) and muscle relaxants (24%).

iii. Initial assessment :

Initial VAS averaged 8/10. The chin-sternum distance at rest was 12.9 cm. In anteflexion of the cervical spine, the chin-sternum distance was 3.2 cm. At extension, this distance was 18.3 cm on average. The average chin-acromion distance was 13.3 cm at right neck rotation, and 13.4 cm at left rotation. At right lateroflexion of the spine, the tragus-acromion distance was 10.7 cm, and at left lateroflexion, this distance was 11.7 cm. The average initial C3-wall distance was 9.9 cm. The initial C7-wall distance was 7.8 cm (Table 1).

<u>**Table 1**</u>: *Initial evaluation data for the 1er group*

	Average	Standard deviation	Minimum	Maximum
EVA pain	8,04/10	1,369	5/10	10/10
Distance between chin and sternum at rest (cm)	12,940	2,9238	4,0	18,0
Distance chin sternum flexion (cm)	3,200	3,3166	0	13,0
Distance chin sternum extension (cm)	18,360	3,6042	10,0	27,0
Distance chin acromion rotation right (cm)	13,360	3,0122	8,0	22,0
Distance chin acromion rotation Left (cm)	13,440	2,7092	9,0	20,0
Distance tragus acromion lateroflexion right (cm)	10,700	2,8831	5,0	16,0
Tragus distance left lateroflexion acromion (cm)	11,740	2,5541	6,0	16,0
Distance C3-Wall (cm)	9,920	3,4269	5,0	18,0
Distance C7-Wall (cm)	7,820	3,0100	3,0	16,0

iv. Evolution :

The VAS after the first 3 acupuncture sessions had risen to 6.4/10. At the end of the treatment, it averaged 2.1/10 (a 73.6% reduction) (Table 2). Eight patients described total disappearance of pain.

***Table 2**: Changes in pain VAS in the 1er group*

EVA pain

	Initial	After 3 sessions	After 6 sessions	At the end of treatment
Average	8,04	6,40	4,64	2,12
Mediane	9,00	7,00	5,00	2,00
Standard deviation	1,369	1,528	1,440	1,965
Minimum	5	4	2	0
Maximum	10	9	8	7

After the first 3 acupuncture sessions, the chin-sternum distance at rest had not changed. It increased at the end of the treatment. After the first 3 acupuncture sessions, at cervical spine anteflexion, the chin-sternum distance had decreased to 1.9 cm. It was 0.6 cm at the end of the treatment. And at extension, after the first 3 acupuncture sessions, this distance had increased to 19.3 cm on average, reaching 20.9 cm at the end of the sessions. (Table 3).

<u>**Table 3**</u>: *Changes in cervical spine flexion and extension amplitudes in 1er group*

Distances (cm)	Average	Spread-type	Minimum	Maximum
Distance between chin and sternum **at rest** initial	12,940	2,9238	4,0	18,0
Chin distance sternum **at rest** After 3eme sessions	12,920	2,4138	5,0	17,0
Chin distance sternum **at rest** After 6eme seance	13,380	2,1079	6,0	16,0
Chin distance sternum **at rest** at the end of the treatment Distance chin	13,220	1,9153	8,0	16,0
sternum **flexion** initial	3,200	3,3166	0	13,0
Distance chin sternum **flexion** After 3eme sessions	1,940	1,5700	0	5,0
Distance chin sternum **flexion** After 6eme session	1,240	1,0618	0	4,0
Distance chin sternum **flexion** at the end of the treatment	0,640	0,7708	0	2,0
Chin distance sternum initial **extension** Distance chin sternum **extension**	18,360	3,6042	10,0	27,0
After 3eme session Distance chin	19,380	3,5422	12,0	29,0
sternum **extension** After 6eme session distance chin	20,400	2,9965	14,0	29,0
sternum **extension** at the	20,960	2,7077	15,0	29,0

end

treatment

After the first 3 acupuncture sessions, the average chin-acromion distance increased to 12.3 cm at right neck rotation and 12.6 cm at left rotation. At the end of the treatment, this distance fell to 10.4 cm in the right-hand rotation of the neck, and 10.8 cm in the left-hand rotation (Table 4).

__Table 4__: Changes in range of rotation of the cervical spine in the 1er group

Distances (cm)	Average	Spread-type	Minimum	Maximum
Distance chin acromion **RDte** initial	13,360	3,0122	8,0	22,0
Distance chin acromion **RDte** After 3eme sessions	12,360	1,8848	8,0	15,0
Distance chin acromion **RDte** After 6eme session	11,300	1,6708	8,0	14,0
Distance chin acromion **RDte** a At the end of treatment	10,420	1,1698	8,0	12,0
Chin distance acromion **RG** initial	13,440	2,7092	9,0	20,0
Chin distance acromion **RG** After 3eme sessions	12,660	2,8458	7,0	19,0
Chin distance acromion **RG** After 6eme session	11,740	2,4669	7,0	18,0
Distance chin acromion **RG** at end of treatment	10,800	1,9149	7,0	16,0

RDte: Rotation to the right, RG: Rotation to the left.

At right lateroflexion of the spine, the tragus-acromion distance was 10 cm after the first 3

11

sessions, and at left lateroflexion, this distance was 10.8 cm. At the end of the sessions, the right lateroflexion of the spine, the tragus-acromion distance was 9.1 cm after the first 3 sessions, and at left lateroflexion, this distance was 9.5 cm (Table 5).

***Table 5**: Changes in lateroflexion amplitudes of the cervical spine in the 1ᵉʳ group*

Distances (cm)	Average	Spread-type	Minimum	Maximum
Distance tragus acromion **ILDte** initial	10,700	2,8831	5,0	16,0
Distance tragus acromion **ILDte** After 3ᵉᵐᵉ sessions	10,020	2,3826	5,0	14,0
Distance tragus acromion **ILDte** After 6ᵉᵐᵉ session	9,460	1,9786	5,0	13,5
Distance tragus acromion **ILDte** at the end of the treatment	9,160	1,7243	5,0	12,0
Distance tragus acromion **ILG** initial	11,740	2,5541	6,0	16,0
Distance tragus acromion **ILG** After 3ᵉᵐᵉ sessions	10,840	2,6129	6,0	16,0
Distance tragus acromion **ILG** After 6ᵉᵐᵉ session	10,060	2,5096	5,0	15,0
Distance tragus acromion **ILG** a la end of treatment	9,560	1,9112	5,0	12,0

ILDte: Lateral tilt or lateroflexion to the right, ILG: Lateral tilt or lateroflexion to the left

After the first 3 acupuncture sessions, the distances C3-wall and C7-wall were 9.2 and 6.7 cm respectively. At the end of the treatment, these distances were 7.7 and 5.9 cm respectively (Table 6).

Table 6*: Trends in cervical spine curvatures in the 1er group*

	Average	Standard deviation	Minimum	Maximum
Distance C3-Wall Initial	9,920	3,4269	5,0	18,0
Distance C3-Wall A3 or MI after 3 sessions	9,260	3,1725	5,0	18,0
Distance C3-Wall after 6 sessions	8,520	2,2055	6,0	15,0
Distance C3-Wall at end of treatment	7,780	2,2917	6,0	14,0
Distance C7-Wall initial	7,820	3,0100	3,0	16,0
Distance C7-Wall after 3 sessions	6,700	2,1213	3,0	10,0
Distance C7-Wall after 6 sessions	6,360	1,8682	3,0	10,0
Distance C7-Wall at end of treatment	5,940	1,7930	3,0	9,0

c. Description of the 2ère group (Mesotherapy Group):

i.   Demographic data :

The 2eme group consisted of 25 patients; 19 women and 6 men. Their average age was 54.9 ±15.9 years [min: 27, max: 82 years]. Seven of them were manual workers, twelve had administrative jobs and the rest were either unemployed or retired.

ii.   Description of symptoms and treatments received:

Neck pain had been evolving for a mean of 5.1 ± 5.8 years [min: 1 month, max: 20 years]. Pain radiated to the upper limb(s) in 72% of cases. The most frequent area of radiation was the C6 root (Figure 3).

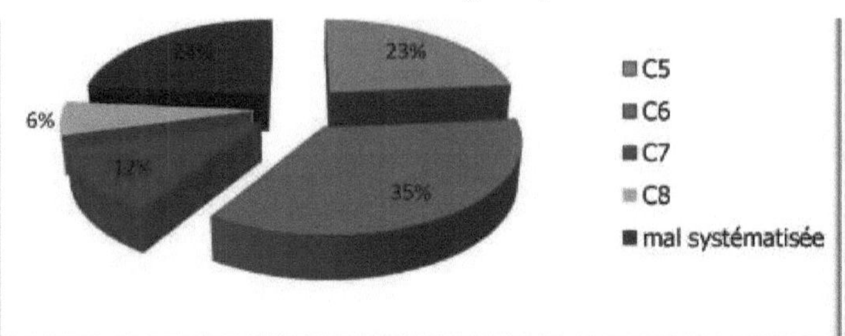

__Figure 3:__ Distribution of cervicalgia irradiation territories in the 2me group

Neck pain was associated with tingling in the hands (68%), headaches (56%), vertigo (28%) and tinnitus (12%).

All the patients in this group had received medical treatment in the last month, and 44% had benefited from rehabilitation in the last 6 months. The drugs most frequently prescribed were analgesics as required (100%), non-steroidal anti-inflammatories (40%) and muscle relaxants (28%).

iii.   Initial assessment :

Initial VAS averaged 7.9/10. The chin-sternum distance at rest was 12.0 cm. In anteflexion of the cervical spine, the chin-sternum distance was 1.2 cm. At extension, this distance was 17.2 cm on average. The average chin-acromion distance was 12.3 cm at right neck rotation, and 12.8 cm at left rotation. In right lateroflexion of the spine, the tragus-acromion distance was 10.4 cm, and

At left lateral flexion, this distance was 11.2 cm. The average initial C3-wall distance was 9.3 cm. The initial C7-wall distance was 7.4 cm (Table 7).

<u>Table 7</u>: Data from the initial evaluation in the 2me group

	Average	Standard deviation	Minimum	Maximum
EVA pain	7,96/10	1,369	5/10	10/10
Distance between chin and sternum at rest (cm)	12,080	2,1922	9,0	18,0
Distance chin sternum flexion (cm)	1,280	2,8250	0	14,0
Distance chin sternum extension (cm)	17,280	2,3188	14,0	22,0
Distance chin acromion rotation right (cm)	12,380	2,1227	7,0	15,0
Distance chin acromion rotation Left (cm) Tragus distance	12,840	1,9670	9,0	17,0
acromion lateroflexion right (cm)	10,440	1,8947	8,0	15,0
Distance tragus acromion left lateroflexion (cm)	11,280	1,6961	8,0	14,0
Distance C3-Wall (cm)	9,560	3,0150	3,0	14,0
Distance C7-Wall (cm)	7,400	1,8200	4,0	11,0

iv. Evolution :

The VAS after the first mesotherapy session had risen to 6.1/10. At the end of the treatment, it averaged 1.5/10 (a reduction of 80.4%) (Table 8). Nine patients described the total disappearance of pain.

**Table 8**: Changes in EVA in the 2me group

EVA pain

	Initial	After 1^e re session	After 2^em th session	At the end of treatment
Average	7,96	6,16	3,64	1,56
Mediane	8,00	6,00	3,00	1,00
Standard deviation	1,369	2,014	2,059	2,311
Minimum	5	2	1	0
Maximum	10	10	9	9

After the first mesotherapy session, the chin-sternum distance at rest had increased to 11.7 cm. It increased at the end of the treatment. After the first 1^e mesotherapy session, at cervical spine anteflexion, the chin-sternum distance had decreased to 0.4 cm. It was 0.2 cm at the end of the treatment. And at extension after the 1st^e mesotherapy session, this distance had increased to 18.4 cm on average, reaching 19.3 cm at the end of the sessions. (Table 9)

Table 9: Changes in cervical spine flexion and extension amplitudes in the 2me group.

Distances (cm)	Average	Standard deviation	Minimum	Maximum
Distance between chin and sternum **at rest** initial	12,080	2,1922	9,0	18,0
Chin distance sternum **at rest** After 1ere session	11,700	2,2314	8,0	18,0
Chin distance sternum **at rest** After 2eme sessions	12,180	2,0355	9,0	18,0
Chin distance sternum **at rest** At the end of the treatment Distance chin	12,540	1,8704	10,0	18,0
sternum **flexion** initial	1,280	2,8250	0	14,0
Distance chin sternum **flexion** After 1ere session	0,440	0,9278	0	4,0
Distance chin sternum **flexion** After 2eme sessions	0,300	0,7360	0	3,0
Distance chin sternum **flexion** At the end of treatment	0,200	0,6455	0	3,0
Chin distance sternum initial **extension** Distance chin sternum **extension** After	17,280	2,3188	14,0	22,0
1ere session Distance chin sternum **extension** After	18,400	2,6964	15,0	24,0
2eme session Distance chin sternum **extension** After	19,120	2,3904	15,0	24,0
sternum **extension** At the	19,320	2,3535	15,0	24,0

end
treatment

After the 1ere mesotherapy session, the average chin-acromion distance increased to 11.3 cm in right neck rotation and 12.1 cm in left rotation. At the end of the treatment, this distance fell to 10.4 cm in right neck rotation and 10.8 cm in left neck rotation (Table 10).

<u>Table 10: Changes in cervical spine range of rotation in the 2me group</u>

Distances (cm)	Average	Standard deviation	Minimum	Maximum
Distance chin acromion **RDte** initial	12,380	2,1227	7,0	15,0
Distance chin acromion **RDte** After 1ere session	11,320	1,9519	7,0	15,0
Chin distance acromion **RDte** After 2eme session	10,960	1,7732	7,0	14,0
Distance chin acromion **RDte** at the end of treatment	10,400	1,4720	7,0	14,0
Chin distance acromion **RG** initial	12,840	1,9670	9,0	17,0
Distance chin acromion **RG** After 1ere session	12,140	1,9393	9,0	17,0
Chin distance acromion **RG** After 2eme sessions	10,820	2,6531	1,0	15,0
Distance chin acromion **RG** at end of treatment	10,800	1,3844	7,0	13,0

RDte: Rotation to the right, RG: Rotation to the left,

At right lateroflexion of the spine, the tragus-acromion distance was 9.8 cm after the 1[ere] session, and at left lateroflexion, this distance was 10.3 cm. At the end of the sessions, in right and left lateroflexion of the spine, the tragus-acromion distance was 9.3 cm bilaterally (Table 11).

<u>***Table 11***</u>***: Changes in lateroflexion amplitudes of the cervical spine in the 2[me] group***

Distances (cm)	Average	Standard deviation	Minimum	Maximum
Tragus distance acromion **ILDte** initial Distance tragus	10,440	1,8947	8,0	15,0
ILDte acromion After 1[ere] session	9,800	1,7078	7,0	14,0
Tragus distance **ILDte** acromion After 2[eme] sessions	9,360	1,3503	7,0	12,0
Tragus distance **ILDte** acromion at the end of treatment	9,340	1,3595	7,0	12,5
Tragus distance acromion **ILG** initial Distance tragus	11,280	1,6961	8,0	14,0
acromion **ILG** Apres 1[ere] seance Distance tragus	10,320	1,2490	9,0	14,0
acromion **ILG** Apres 2[eme] seance Distance tragus	10,000	2,5083	7,0	19,5
ILG acromion at the end of treatment	9,360	1,2871	7,0	12,0

ILDte: Lateral tilt or lateroflexion on the right, ILG: lateral inclination or lateroflexion a left

After the 1[ere] mesotherapy session, the distances C3-wall and C7-wall were 8.9 and 6.9 cm respectively. At the end of the treatment, these distances were 7.8 and 6.7 cm respectively

(Table 12).

***Table 12**: Trends in cervical spine curvatures in the 2me group*

Distances (cm)	Average	Standard deviation	Minimum	Maximum
Distance C3-Wall Initial	9,560	3,0150	3,0	14,0
Distance C3-Wall A3 or MI after 1ere session	8,960	2,5410	3,0	13,0
Distance C3-Wall after 2eme session	8,220	2,3456	3,0	13,0
Distance C3-Wall a la end of treatment	7,860	1,9975	3,0	12,0
Distance C7-Initial wall	7,400	1,8200	4,0	11,0
Distance C7-Wall after 1ere session	6,980	1,5033	4,0	10,0
Distance C7-Wall after 2eme session	6,880	1,3940	4,0	10,0
Distance C7-Wall at end of treatment	6,760	1,3317	4,0	9,0

2] **Analytical study :**

a. **Comparability of the two groups :**

i. Demographic data :

There was no significant difference between the two groups in terms of gender (p=0.37) (Figure 4).

Gender comparison between the two groups

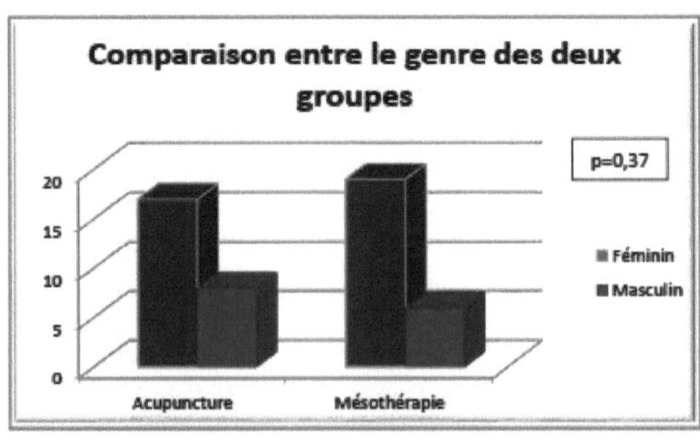

Figure 4   *Gender comparison of the two groups*

There was no significant difference between the two groups in terms of mean age (p=0.54).

Similarly, there was no statistically significant difference in terms of profession between patients in the two groups (p=0.24) (Figure 5).

Comparison between occupations in the 2 groups

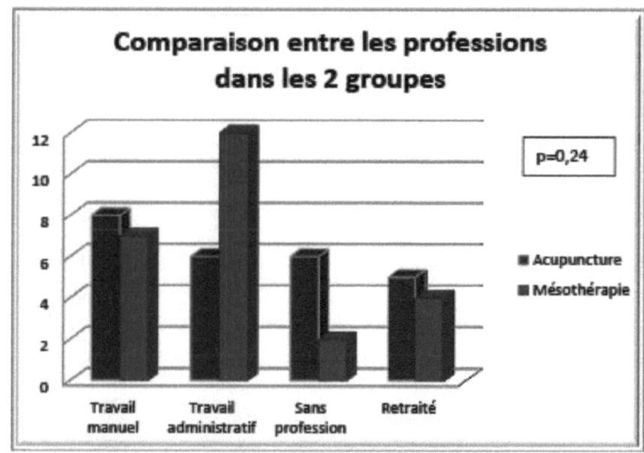

Figure 5: Comparison of occupations in the 2 groups

ii. Description of symptoms:

We will focus on the age of symptoms. There was no significant difference between the two groups in terms of the age of the pain (p=0.28).

iii. Treatment received :

There was a significant difference between the two groups in terms of drug intake (p=0.025). In detailing drug intake, this significance only concerned analgesics, and not NSAIDs or muscle relaxants (Table 13). Analgesics as required were prescribed to all patients in the 2me group.

Table 13: Comparison of drug intake in the two groups

	Acupuncture Group Nb (%)	Group Mesotherapy Nb (%)	p
Analgesics as required	20 (44,4)	25 (55,6)	**0,025**
NSAIDS	8 (44,4)	10 (55,6)	0,384
Muscle relaxants	6 (46,2)	7 (53,8)	0,500
Taking medication Whatever it is	20 (44,4)	25 (55,6)	**0,025**

There was no significant difference between the number of patients in the 2 groups who had received functional rehabilitation in the 6 months prior to treatment (p=0.128).

21

b. <u>Comparison between revolution de LEVA :</u>

There was a significant difference only in the VAS after the 6me acupuncture session and the 2^{ète} mesotherapy session, with a more rapid improvement in pain in the 2me group (Table 14). There was no difference between the VAS at the end of the treatment.

<u>Table 14</u>: Comparison of the evolution of EVA

	EVA pain		
	Group Acupuncture	Group Mesotherapy	p
Initial EVA	8,04	7,96	0,83
EVA A3 or MI	6,40	6,16	0,63
EVA A6 or M2	4,64	3,64	**0,05**
EVA at the end of treatment	2,12	1,56	0,36

c. <u>Comparison of cervical spine amplitudes :</u>

At initial assessment, the only significant difference between the two groups was in the chin-sternum distance at flexion, which was less in the 2me group (Table 15). Moreover, this advantage of the 2me group persisted throughout the treatment.

For the other ranges of movement of the cervical spine, only the chin-sternum distance at extension at the end of treatment showed a significant difference between the two groups, with a greater improvement for the 1er group (Table 15).

<u>**Table 15**</u>: *Comparison of changes in cervical spine extension and flexion amplitudes*

Distances (cm)	Acupuncture Group	Mesotherapy Group	p
Chin distance sternum at **rest** initial	12,940	12,080	0,24
Chin distance sternum at **rest** After A3 or MI	12,920	11,700	0,07
Chin distance sternum at **rest** After A6 or M2	13,380	12,180	**0,04**
Chin distance sternum at **rest** a At the end of treatment	13,220	12,540	0,21
Chin distance sternum **flexion** initial	3,200	1,280	**0,03**
Chin distance sternum **flexion** After A3 or MI	1,940	0,440	**<0,001**
Chin distance sternum **flexion** After A6 or M2	1,240	0,300	**0,001**
Chin distance sternum **flexion** at end of treatment	0,640	0,200	**0,03**
Chin distance sternum **extension** initial	18,360	17,280	0,21
Chin distance sternum **extension** After A3 or MI	19,380	18,400	0,27
Chin distance sternum **extension** After A6 or M2	20,400	19,120	0,10

Chin distance sternum **extension** at the end of treatment	20,960	19,320	**0,02**

A3 : 3^{em} e acupuncture session, A6 : 6^{em} e acupuncture session, MI : First mesotherapy session, M2 : 2^{em} e mesotherapy session

There was no significant difference between the two groups in the range of rotation of the cervical spine during revolution. (Table 16)

Tableau 16: ***Comparison of***
the evolution of
cervical spine rotation amplitudes

Distances (cm)	Acupuncture Group	Mesotherapy Group	p
Distance chin acromion **RDte** initial	13,360	12,380	0,19
Distance chin acromion **RDte** After A3 or MI	12,360	11,320	0,06
Distance chin acromion **RDte** After A6 or M2	11,300	10,960	0,48
Distance chin acromion **RDte** a la end of treatment	10,420	10,400	0,95
Distance chin acromion **RG** initial	13,440	12,840	0,37
Distance chin acromion **RG** After A3 or MI	12,660	12,140	0,45
Distance chin acromion **RG** After A6 or M2	11,740	10,820	0,21
Distance chin acromion **RG** to end treatment	10,800	10,800	1,00

RDte: Rotation to the right, RG: Rotation to the left, A3:3eme acupuncture session, A6: 6eme acupuncture session, MI: 1ere mesotherapy session, M2: 2eme mesotherapy session

There was no significant difference between the two groups for the amplitudes of lateroflexion of the cervical spine during revolution. (Table 17)

Tableau 17: ***Comparison of***

the evolution of

the amplitudes of lateroflexion of the cervical spine

Distances (cm)	Acupuncture Group	Mesotherapy Group	p
Distance tragus acromion **ILDte** initial	10,700	10,440	0,70
Distance tragus acromion **ILDte** After A3 or MI	10,020	9,800	0,70
Distance tragus acromion **ILDte** After A6 or M2	9,460	9,360	0,83
Distance tragus acromion **ILDte** at end of treatment	9,160	9,340	0,68
Distance tragus acromion initial **ILG**	11,740	11,280	0,45
Distance tragus acromion **ILG** After A3 or MI	10,840	10,320	0,37
Distance tragus acromion **ILG** After A6 or M2	10,060	10,000	0,93
Distance tragus acromion **ILG** at end of treatment	9,560	9,360	0,66

ILDte: lateral inclination or lateroflexion to the right, ILG: lateral inclination or lateroflexion to the left, A3:3[eme] acupuncture session, A6: 6[eme] acupuncture session, M1: 1[ere] mesotherapy session, M2: 2[eme] mesotherapy session

d. Comparison of the revolution of the cervical spine arches

There was no significant difference between the two groups in terms of the attitude of the cervical spine in the sagittal plane (Table 18). In fact, there was a decrease in anteprojection of the cervical spine in all patients, regardless of the treatment method chosen.

Tableau 18: *Comparison between arrow revolutions of the cervical spine*

Distances (cm)	Acupuncture Group	Mesotherapy Group	p
Distance C3-Wall Initial	9,920	9,560	0,69
Distance C3-Wall A3 or MI after A3 or MI	9,260	8,960	0,71
Distance C3-Wall after A6 or M2	8,520	8,220	0,64
Distance C3-Wall at the end treatment	7,780	7,860	0,89
Distance C7-Initial wall	7,820	7,400	0,55
Distance C7-Wall after A3 or MI	6,700	6,980	0,59
Distance C7-Wall after A6 or M2	6,360	6,880	0,27
Distance C7-Wall at the end treatment	5,940	6,760	**0,07**

A3: 3eme acupuncture session, A6: 6eme acupuncture session, MI: 1ere mesotherapy session, M2: 2eme mesotherapy session

4 Discussion

Chronic neck pain is a frequent complaint in our clinics. They are treated in a multidisciplinary way, combining medical treatment and rehabilitation. This treatment often takes a long time, sometimes with only moderately satisfactory results. In order to relieve patients' pain more quickly, or even more effectively, the practitioner uses so-called complementary therapies, such as acupuncture or mesotherapy.

Our study showed that mesotherapy provided faster pain relief for patients, but that at the end of treatment the two methods were equivalent. Acupuncture resulted in better cervical spine extension at the end of treatment.

In the following chapters, we will discuss the contribution of each of the techniques to cervicarthrosis or chronic neck pain. We will then compare the two techniques, based on our results and those of the literature. Finally, we will attempt to draw up some recommendations.

1] <u>The contribution of acupuncture in the treatment of chronic neck pain :</u>

In our study, acupuncture improved cervical spine pain and amplitude in patients in the 1er group. In fact, 8 out of 25 patients described a total disappearance of pain at the end of the treatment, with an average VAS of 2.1/10 for this group. We also noted an increase in the flexibility of cervical spine movements in all planes of space: flexion, extension, right and left rotations and lateral tilts. A reduction in anteprojection of the cervical spine was also noted.

Most of the Tunisian studies on this subject were carried out in the same acupuncture department of the CHU Mongi Slim La Marsa, as part of a dissertation for the end of a certificate of further studies [15-18]. They assessed pain using the VAS and found, like ours, a reduction in pain at the end of the treatment (Table 19). The same was true for spinal stiffness, which improved significantly [15,16,18]. Guermazi's study also noted a rapid improvement in vertigo from the end of the 3eme session, and in paresthesia from the end of the 6eme session [15]. In Haddad's study, the variation in VAS was not correlated with age, sex, professional profile, the age of the neck pain or the patient's belief in the efficacy of acupuncture [16]. The results were maintained one month after the end of treatment in Zgolli's study [17]. The main limitation of these studies was the absence of a control group. And as far as the methodology was concerned, these different studies only assessed the flexibility of the cervical spine by the chin-sternum distance during flexion [15-17]. Furthermore, these studies did not assess the efficacy of acupuncture in isolation. In fact, it was combined with either electropuncture, cervical traction, or both. This makes comparison between the various Tunisian studies, including our own, approximate.

<u>Table 19</u>: Changes in VAS in Tunisian studies

	Year	Number of	Average age	Initial EVA	EVA	VAS at the

	year	patients	(years)	EVA	after 3rd seance	after 6th seance	end of treatment
Guermazi [15]	2014	35	54	8,0	5,2	3,1	1,6
Haddad [16]	2007	30	54,1 ±10,6	7,1	NM	4,4	2,0
Zgolli [17]	2004	50	51,9 ±11,7	7,1	NM	4,4	1,8
Tlili [18]	2003	21	NM [min:36, max:78]	5,8	4,2	3,9	4,0
Our study	2015	25	57,5 ±13,7	8,0	6,4	4,6	2,1

NM: not mentioned

The international literature, especially that from Asia [19-27], is much richer than that from Tunisia. The results of the studies were rather encouraging.

In a recent randomised controlled study, the VAS for pain fell from 5.3/10 initially, to 3.4 at the end of treatment, and to 2.8/10 3 months after the end of treatment (p=0.04) [26]. Another Spanish study found similar results with VAS at baseline, at the end of treatment and 6 months after the end of treatment respectively at 6.8/10, 4.2/10 and 4.1/10 [28]. Another British cohort study, involving 172 patients who had received acupuncture treatment with or without a "conventional" treatment (medication, rehabilitation, etc.) for chronic neck pain, found that 68% of them reported an improvement of at least 50%, with 14/172 patients reporting total disappearance of pain [29].

Acupuncture has been shown to provide more than pain relief in the treatment of chronic neck pain. In fact, in a German multicentre randomised controlled trial published in 2006, an assessment of quality of life using the Bullinger and Kirchberger SF36 score [30], in patients who had received acupuncture for chronic neck pain, showed a significant improvement in the score compared with the control group [31]. This study also demonstrated that at 3 and 6 months after the end of treatment, the acupuncture group retained its superiority in terms of pain and quality of life.

Although the majority of studies were positive, a 2004 critical analysis of the literature called these results into question [32]. It pointed the finger at the small numbers involved in randomised controlled trials. Therapeutically, it highlighted the fact that acupuncture was rarely used alone (cervical traction, electropuncture, moxibustion).

The same applies to our study. One of its main limitations is that it did not use acupuncture alone in the treatment of chronic neck pain. In fact, 80% had received medical treatment in the month prior to going into labour (or were still receiving it), and 64% had benefited from rehabilitation in the last 6 months. As for the therapeutic protocol, acupuncture was always combined with electropuncture. Another shortcoming of our work was that we did not assess the patients at a distance from the treatment, in the medium and long term. And finally, 25 patients is not a large number to be able to really judge the effectiveness of this therapy.

In our study, no side-effects related to acupuncture were reported. The good tolerance of acupuncture has been confirmed by several studies [28,33,34]. However, some publications have mentioned minor adverse effects such as bruising, subcutaneous hematoma and bleeding from the puncture site [28,35-37]. Patients with blood disorders were not systematically included in our work, which may explain the fact that we did not note any particular incidents. In another study, 3 patients out of 88 experienced discomfort during treatment [26]. This incident, known *DISCUSSION* in Chinese medicine as "needle sickness", can be prevented by performing the puncture in a supine position, in a calm environment and by reassuring the patient. In a study of the adverse effects of acupuncture on 34,000 patients in the United Kingdom, MacPherson found a rate of 1.3%o of minor incidents, without observing any major accidents [38].

2] **The contribution of mesotherapy in the treatment of chronic neck pain:**

In our study, mesotherapy improved cervical spine pain and amplitude in patients in the 2eme group. Indeed, 9 out of 25 patients described a total disappearance of pain at the end of treatment, with an average VAS of 1.5/10 for this group. We also noted an increase in the flexibility of cervical spine movements in all planes of space: flexion, extension, right and left rotations and lateral tilts. A reduction in anteprojection of the cervical spine was also noted.

Tunisian studies dealing with mesotherapy and chronic neck pain are rare. The study most similar to ours was carried out in the same centre, Institut Mohamed Kassab D'orthopedie de Ksar Said, and published in 1998 [39]. It involved 35 patients treated for chronic neck pain, with an average age of 49.7 years [min: 28, max: 67 years]. The patients had previously received analgesic treatment, non-steroidal anti-inflammatory drugs, muscle relaxants and had followed an adapted rehabilitation programme. 10 patients were very satisfied, with complete regression of their symptoms. 19 patients improved with a reduction in NSAID consumption but required maintenance sessions. 6 reported no improvement. The mean follow-up was 17 months, with extremes of 1 month and 3^{1} /2 years. No side effects were noted. The limitation of this study is that it did not specify the evaluation methods used, or the frequency of these evaluations. Its size was limited, and the results were not compared. *DISCUSSION* a control group. And finally, mesotherapy was not used on its own, but in combination with a so-called conventional treatment.

Other Tunisian studies have dealt globally with the contribution of mesotherapy in musculoskeletal disorders in general and in certain pathologies in particular (scapulalgia, gonarthrosis, common lumbago, etc.). In a study published in 2014, on a group of patients suffering from musculoskeletal pain (including 14% neck pain), who had received 4 weeks of mesotherapy treatment, 57.2% of them were satisfied, with 11% of patients no longer suffering from pain [13].

The international literature is also sparse. Indeed, few published works have dealt with the contribution of mesotherapy in neck pain. An Italian publication dating from 1991, based on 20 patients suffering from cervicobrachial neuralgia, compared two groups: 1er treated with TENS (Transcutaneous Electrical Nerve Stimulation) and 2eme with mesotherapy combined with TENS [40]. It concluded that the combination was superior in terms of pain and speed of improvement. Two other multicentre Italian studies had investigated the effect of mesotherapy on certain painful osteoarticular disorders, including neck pain, with injections combining NSAIDs ± procaine and muscle relaxants, at a rate of one session per week for 21 days, for up to 984 patients (but without a control group) [41,42]. They found a reduction in pain of up to 87% in patients with neck pain. In a 2012 publication, the Italian Society of Mesotherapy recognised the efficacy and good tolerance of this treatment (a combination of muscle relaxant and NSAID) in the treatment of musculoskeletal pain [43]. She emphasised the lack of systemic adverse effects of NSAIDs using this technique. And she emphasised the fact that this therapy was all the more effective when combined with standard treatment based on oral analgesics and rehabilitation.

As with the acupuncture group, one of the limitations of this work on mesotherapy is that we did not use this technique alone. In fact, all the patients were taking analgesics on demand and 44% had benefited from rehabilitation during the previous 6 months. Nor did we carry out a remote evaluation, and a population of 25 patients is too small to be able to make a real assessment of the effectiveness of this therapy. Another obstacle to comparison between the various studies and with our own is the fact that the therapeutic protocol itself is not well codified. In fact, apart from the exact number of sessions and the total duration of treatment, almost every study used different products for the injections, sometimes alone or in combination (Table 20).

Table 20*: *Different mesotherapy treatment protocols and indications

Study	Year	Indication	Products used	Number of sessions and duration of treatment
Palermo [40]	1991	Cervicobrachial neuralgia	Lidocaine Muscle relaxants	4 sessions 20 days

Parrini [44]	2002	Acute lumbosciatica	Acetyl salicylic acid	1 single session
Monticone [45]	2004	Low back pain (sacroiliac dysfunction)	NSAIDS	8 sessions 28 days
Costantino [46]	2011	Acute low back pain	Lidocaine Ketoprofene	5 sessions 13 days
Di Cesare [47]	2011	Chronic low back pain	Lidocaine	4 sessions 28 days
Narvarte [48]	2011	Mechanical scapulalgia	Thiocolchicoside Diazepam Buflomedil Piroxicam	1 to 18 sessions Duration NM
Our study	2015	Chronic neck pain	Lidocaine Thiocolchicoside Ketoprofene	3 sessions 21 days

NM: not mentioned, NSAID: Non-steroidal anti-inflammatory drug

In our study, no side-effects related to mesotherapy were reported. And despite the almost unanimous agreement in the literature on the good tolerance of this technique, some studies have noted a few incidents. Transient and reversible cutaneous reactions such as tingling, allergic reactions, ecchymosis and urticaria have sometimes been noted [48]. These reactions have been attributed either to poor injection technique or to the products used themselves [43]. Rare cases of skin infections have been reported [49-51]. In our work, we followed rigorous hygiene rules, disinfecting the skin before injections with 70° alcohol.

3] <u>Comparison between acupuncture and mesotherapy in the treatment of chronic neck pain :</u>

Our study showed that mesotherapy provided significantly faster pain relief for patients, but that at the end of treatment the two methods were equivalent. Acupuncture resulted in better cervical spine extension at the end of treatment. There was no significant difference between the two groups in terms of the attitude of the cervical spine in the sagittal plane.

To our knowledge, there is no publication comparable to ours in either local or international literature.

However, an Italian work by Di Cesare, published in 2011, may be relevant in this context. The author compared trigger point mesotherapy and acupuncture point mesotherapy in the treatment of chronic low back pain [47]. This was a randomised controlled study with two groups. The 1[er] group, 29 patients with a mean age of 52.5 ± 12.1 years, received Lidocaine-based mesotherapy at 18 trigger points identified according to the method of

Travell and Simons [52,53]. The 2eme group, 33 patients with a mean age of 52.5 ± 12.9 years, had received Lidocaine-based mesotherapy at the following acupuncture points: VB34, VB41, VB 30, V60, V31, V52, DM3, R4, TR5 and dorsal Ashi points. Both groups received one session per week for 4 weeks. Pain was assessed using the visual analogue scale (VAS) and the verbal analogue scale. Functional impact was assessed using the Roland Morris Disability Scale Questionnaire (RMQ) [54] and the Oswestry Low Back Pain Disability Questionnaire (ODQ) [55]. The results showed that in the group receiving acupuncture point mesotherapy, patients reported a significantly better improvement in terms of pain and functional gain than the 1er group. This result was maintained 4 weeks after stopping treatment. The author noted adverse effects in only 4 patients in the 2eme group, between the 1ere and 2eme sessions, which disappeared before the 3eme session. The author described neck pain as minimal.

Comparing the effectiveness of the two techniques, as described in the previous chapters, we can see from the literature that both methods are promising. As far as adverse effects are concerned, the incidents encountered with acupuncture appear to be more benign. Mesotherapy also imposed a restriction of indication, that of drug allergies, sometimes encountered with NSAIDs.

However, when we compared the therapeutic protocol, we found that mesotherapy was less restrictive for the patient, with only one weekly session compared with 3 for acupuncture.

4] **Recommendations:**

The main recommendations concern the methodology to be followed for future work. It would be interesting to compare the two therapeutic methods in randomised controlled trials with larger numbers. With regard to the therapeutic protocol, it would also be judicious to standardise the methods. In fact, acupuncture was combined with cervical traction, electropuncture, cupping etc... And similarly for mesotherapy, the products and injection techniques varied from one study to another. We also propose to evaluate the two methods in the medium and long term.

Furthermore, mesotherapy remains an empirical technique in Tunisia, in the absence of training recognised by the Tunis Faculty of Medicine. We propose the creation of a diploma within the Faculty to regularise the activity of doctors practising mesotherapy.

In conclusion, we leave it up to the practitioner to choose the complementary medicine method that he is most familiar with and/or has the easiest access to. He must know how to indicate one or the other depending on the patient's potential adherence to the sessions (numerous for acupuncture, and fewer for mesotherapy). He must also be aware of the contraindications for each treatment (for example, wearing a pacemaker for electropuncture, an allergy to NSAIDs for mesotherapy, hemostasis disorders for both treatments, etc.).

5 Conclusions

Chronic neck pain is a frequent reason for consultation, both in 1ere line facilities and in specialist consultations. It is a public health problem because of its disabling and recurrent nature, and its cost to the community. They require multidisciplinary treatment, combining medication and rehabilitation. In order to relieve patients' pain more quickly, or even more effectively, practitioners use so-called complementary therapies, such as acupuncture and mesotherapy. Acupuncture is a therapy based on traditional Chinese medicine, which dates back 4,000 years. Mesotherapy is a relatively recent technique, introduced by Dr Pistor in the 50s. Its benefits as an adjunctive therapy in the treatment of musculoskeletal pain, particularly chronic neck pain, are well recognised. The aims of this study were to assess the clinical effectiveness of mesotherapy and acupuncture as adjunctive treatments for mechanical neck pain of degenerative origin, and to compare the short-term efficacy of these two therapies.

This was a prospective study which took place between August 2015 and December of the same year. It involved 50 patients suffering from neck pain, divided equally into two groups: the 1er group who consulted the acupuncture department of the Mongi Slim Hospital in La Marsa, and the 2eme group who consulted the Physical Medicine and Functional Rehabilitation department of the Mohamed Kassab Orthopaedic Institute. On inclusion, and after informed oral consent, all patients were questioned about the intensity of their neck pain (assessed by the visual analogue scale VAS), the age of their symptoms, and whether or not they had neuralgia. This 1er consultation also provided an opportunity to assess the mobility of the cervical spine (chin-sternum distances for flexion and extension, chin-acromion distances for right and left rotation and ear-acromion tragus distances for right and left lateral tilt) and to look for postural abnormalities (distances between the spinous processes of C3 and C7 and the plumb line (or wall)).

Patients in the 1er group, who consulted the acupuncture department at the CHU Mongi Slim in La Marsa, received a prescription for 10 sessions at a rate of 3 sessions per week. This prescription may or may not have been combined with conventional medical treatment (medication, rehabilitation, use of a neck brace, etc.). The acupuncture treatment involved a combination of local points and standard remote points for neck pain, Ashi points, and points on the path of the irradiations. Electrical stimulation of the puncture needles was also applied. A clinical evaluation, including all the items from the initial clinical examination, as well as a pain VAS was carried out after the 3eme and 6eme sessions (A3, A6), and at the end of the treatment (1 week after the last session) (A10).

Patients in the 2eme group, who consulted the Physical Medicine and Functional Rehabilitation department of the Mohamed Kassab Orthopaedic Institute, were prescribed 3 mesotherapy sessions, one per week. This prescription may or may not have been combined with conventional medical treatment (medication, rehabilitation, use of a neck brace, etc.). The mesotherapy treatment consisted of a combination of 2 techniques: a series of deep intra-dermal point-by-point IDP injections into the painful areas of a mixture of : Lidocaine, thiocolchicoside and ketoprofen using a 4 mm needle, and a superficial intradermal coating using a mixture of Lidocaine and thiocolchicoside using a 13 mm needle. A clinical evaluation, including all the items from the initial clinical examination, as well as a pain VAS was carried out after the 1eme and 2eme sessions (M1, M2), and one week after the 3eme session; the end of treatment (M3).

Data was entered and analysed using SPSS® 17.01 (Statistical Package for Social Sciences, SPSS Inc, Chicago, Illinois). Graphs were produced using Excel® 12.0 (Microsoft Office 2007, Microsoft Corporation, Washington). A systematic review of the literature was also carried out. We selected English- and French-language articles published between 1976 and 2016 by consulting the Medline and Google Scholar databases. The keywords used alone or in combination were as follows: Acupuncture, Mesotherapy, mesotherapie, cervicalgies chroniques, chronic neck pain. We also consulted the results of Tunisian studies, which mainly took the form of master's or CEC dissertations, as well as oral or poster communications.

The total number of patients was 50, with a mean age of 56.2 ±13.7 years. There were 36 women and 14 men. Our patients had been suffering from neck pain for a mean of 6.1 years [min: 1 month, max: 25 years].

The average age in the 1er group was 57.5 ± 13.7 years, and 54.9 ± 15.9 years in the 2eme group (p=0.54). There were 17 women and 8 men in the 1er group, and 19 women and 6 men in the 2eme group (p=0.37). Similarly, there was no statistically significant difference in terms of occupation between patients in the two groups (p=0.24). Pain had been evolving for a mean of 7.1 ± 6.7 years in the 1er group and 5.1 ± 5.8 years in the 2eme group (p=0.28). In the acupuncture group, pain radiated to the upper limb(s) in 64% of cases. In the other group, radiation was present in 72%. 80% of patients in the 1er group had received medical treatment in the last month, and 64% had benefited from rehabilitation in the last 6 months. All patients in the 2eme group had received medication in the last month (p=0.025), and 44% had received rehabilitation in the last 6 months (p=0.128). The drugs most frequently prescribed were analgesics as required (80% for the 1er group and 100% for the 2eme group; p=0.025), non-steroidal anti-inflammatory drugs (NSAIDs) (32% for the 1er group and 40% for the 2eme group; p=0.38) and muscle relaxants (24% for the 1er group and 28% for the 2eme group; p=0.50).

The average initial pain VAS was 8/10 in the acupuncture group and 7.9/10 in the mesotherapy group (p=0.83). For the other data from the initial clinical examination, there was only one significant difference between the two groups. This concerned the chin-sternum distance in flexion. We therefore did not base our conclusions on this parameter.

In our study, acupuncture improved cervical spine pain and amplitude in patients in the 1er group. This is because,

CONCLUSIONS 8 out of 25 patients described a total disappearance of pain at the end of treatment, with a mean VAS of 2.1/10 for this group. In our study, mesotherapy improved cervical spine pain and amplitude in patients in the 2me group. Indeed, 9 out of 25 patients described a total disappearance of pain at the end of the treatment, with an average VAS of 1.5/10 for this group. We also noted an increase in the flexibility of cervical spine movements in all planes of space: flexion, extension, right and left rotations and lateral tilts in both groups. A reduction in anteprojection of the cervical spine was also noted in all patients, all methods combined.

There was only a significant difference in the VAS after the 6eme acupuncture session and the 2me mesotherapy session, with a faster improvement in pain for the 2me group (p=0.05). However, at the end of the treatment, the two methods were equivalent (no significant difference).

Acupuncture resulted in a better range of extension of the cervical spine at the end of the treatment. The chin-sternum distance at extension was 20.9 cm for the 1er group at the end of treatment, and 19.3 cm for the 2me group (p=0.02).

There was no significant difference between the two groups in terms of the attitude of the cervical spine in the sagittal plane. In fact, there was a reduction in anteprojection of the cervical spine in all patients, regardless of the treatment method chosen.

In comparing the efficacy of the two techniques, whether through our work or the results found in the literature, we found that both methods appeared to be promising. However, given the insufficient number of studies involving mesotherapy in Tunisia, we recommend more work before deciding on the superiority of one method over the other. When we also compared the therapeutic protocol, we noted that mesotherapy was less restrictive for the patient, with only one weekly session compared with 3 for acupuncture. We also recommend greater standardisation of protocols, especially for mesotherapy. We also suggest that future studies compare the efficacy of the two treatment methods over the medium and long term.

In conclusion, we leave it to the practitioner to choose the complementary medicine method that he is most familiar with and/or has the easiest access to. He must know how to indicate one or the other depending on the patient's potential adherence to the sessions (numerous for acupuncture, and fewer but involving the injection of medication for mesotherapy). He must also be aware of the contraindications for each (for example: wearing a pace maker in the case of electropuncture, an allergy to NSAIDs in the case of mesotherapy, hemostasis disorders in the case of both, etc.).

References

1] Hildingsson MC, Nilsson M. The prevalence of neck pain: a population-based study for northern Sweden. Acta Orthop Scand. 2002;73:455-9

2] Vincent K. Systematic analysis of the effectiveness of manual therapeutics in common neck pain. Rev Rhum. 2013 ;80:503-511.

3] Vital JM, Lavignolle BV, Pointillart O, Gille, De Seze M. Cervicalgia commune et nevralgies cervicobrachiale. Encyclopedie Medico-Chirurgicale (Elsevier Masson SAS, Paris), 15-831-A-10, 2004

4] Manh Don N, Phankim-Koupernik M. And acupuncture? (pp. 173-178). In: de Seze S, Ryckewaert A, Kahn M-F, Guerin CL, editors. I'Actualite Rhumatologique 1971. Paris: Expansion Scientifique; 1971.

5] Ernst E. Complementary and alternative medicine in rheumatology. Bailliere's Clinical Rheumatology. 2000;14:731-49.

6] Sandberg M, Lundeberg T, Lindberg L, Gerdle B. Effects of acupuncture on skin and muscle blood flow in healthy subjects. European Journal of Applied Physiology. 2003;90(1-2):114-9.

7] Sato A, Sato Y, Schmidt R. The impact of somatosensory input on autonomic functions. Heidelberg: Springer-Verlag; 1997.

8] Zhao Z. Neural mechanisms underlying acupuncture analgesia. Neurobiology. 2008;85:355-75.

9] Lundeberg T, Ekholm J. Pain - from periphery to brain. Journal of the Acupuncture Association of Chartered Physiotherapists. 2001:13-9.

10] Bradnam L. A proposed clinical reasoning model for western acupuncture. Journal of the Acupuncture Association of Chartered Physiotherapists. 2007:21-30.

11] Pistor M. Un défi therapeutique: la mesotherapie. 3eme edition. Paris: Maloine, 1979, 272 p.

12] Lavignolle B, de Seze M, de Boysson A, Lavignolle V, Fourquet M, Jeanmaire Y, et al. Mesotherapy in the treatment of projected pain in degenerative spinal pathology. Randomised controlled studies versus infiltrations. In:1er Congres national de Mesotherapie, Paris22-23 mars 2003.

13] Boudokhane S, El Mtaoua S, Salah S, Migaou H, Aoud W, Elmay W, et al. Interet de la mesotherapie dans le traitement des douleurs musculo-squelettiques en MPR. Annals of Physical and Rehabilitation Medicine. 2014;57S:e202-e211

14] Gouilly P, Petitdant B, Braun R, Royer A, Cordier JP. Cervical spine assessment. EMC (Elsevier Masson SAS, Paris), Kinesitherapie-Medecine physique-Readaptation, 26-008-G-10, 2009

15] Guermazi S. Contribution of acupuncture associated with cervical traction in the treatment of chronic neck pain. [Memoire] Acupuncture, 2014, Tunis.

16] Haddad A. Treatment of osteoarthritic neck pain by acupuncture, apropos of 30 cases. [Memoire] Acupuncture, 2007, Tunis.

17] Zgolli S. Efficacy of acupuncture in the treatment of cervicarthrosis in 50 cases. [Memoire] Acupuncture, 2004, Tunis.

18] Tlili A. Place de l'acupuncture dans le traitement des cervicalgies. [Memoire] Acupuncture, 2003, Tunis.

19] Liu MJ, Mu JP, Zheng S, Ren CJ. Efficacy observation on cervical spondylosis of nerve root type treated by the warm needling at Jiaji (EX-B 2) and tapping with plum-blossom needle. World Jour of Acupuncture Moxibustion. 2013 ;23:6-10.

20] Wang C, Wu Y, Zhang J, Huang C. Observation on Efficacy of Acupoint Injection Combined with Traction for Cervical Radiculopathy. Journal of Acupunture and Tuina Science. 2011;9:380-83.

21] Yi-Qun MI. Clinical Study on Electro-acupuncture plus Traction in Treating Cervical Disk Extrusion in 100 Cases. Journal of Acupunture and Tuina Science. 2006;4:227-9.

22] Wu L, Yang XZ. Clinical Observation on Treatment of Cervical Spondylosis with Acupuncture plus Traction. Journal of Acupunture and Tuina Science. 2005;3:39-41.

23] Qian Xi. Treatment of cervical spondylotic radiculopathy: acupuncture at neck Jiaji points and blood-letting puncture with the plum-blossom needle. World Jour of Acup-Moxibus. 2012;22:1-4.

24] Zhang ZS, Chen QI. Treatment of Cervical Spondylosis in 73 Cases by Warm Acupuncture plus Traction. Journal of Acupunture and Tuina Science. 2005;3:46-7.

25] Zhang XY, Yao GZ. Treatment of 40 Cases of Cervical Vertigo by Acupuncture. Journal of Acupunture and Tuina Science. 2003;1(2):41-2.

26] Liang Z, Zhu X, Yanga X, Fua W, Lu A. Assessment of a traditional acupuncture therapy for chronic neck pain: A pilot randomized controlled study. Complementary Therapies in Medicine. 2011;19S:S26-S32

27] Itoh K, Katsumi Y, Hirota S, Kitakoji H. Randomized trial of trigger point acupuncture compared with other acupuncture for treatment of chronic neck pain. Complementary Therapies in Medicine. 2007;15:172-17.

28] Vas J, Perea-Milla E, Mendez C, Navarro SC, Rubio JML, Brioso M, Obrero IG. Efficacy and safety of acupuncture for chronic uncomplicated neck pain: A randomised controlled study. Pain. 2006;126:245-55.

29] Blossfeldt P. Acupuncture for chronic neck pain - a cohort study in an NHS pain clinic. Acupuncture In Medicine. 2004;22(3):146-151.

30] Bullinger M, Kirchberger I. SF-36 Fragebogen zum Gesundheitszustand. Gottingen: Hogrefe; 1998.

31] Witt CM, Jena S, Brinkhaus B, Liecker B, Wegscheider K, Willich NS. Acupuncture for patients with chronic neck pain. Pain. 2006;125:98-106.

32] Beaudreuil J, Gallou JJ. Acupuncture and chronic neck pain: a critical review of the literature. Rev Rhu. 2004;71:721-3.

33] Berman BM, Langenberg P, Hochberg M. Effectiveness of Acupuncture as Adjunctive Therapy in Osteoarthritis of the knee. Ann Intern Med. 2004;141:901-10.

34] Tukmachi E, Jubb R, Dempsey E, Jones P. The effect of acupuncture on the symptoms of knee osteoarthritis- an open randomized controlled study. Acup Med. 2004;22:14-22.

35] Foster NE, Thomas E, Barlas P. Acupuncture as an adjunct to exercise based physiotherapy for osteoarthritis of the knee: randomized controlled trial. BMJ. 2007;335:436-40.

36] Scharf HP, Mansmann U, Streitberger Kl. Acupuncture and Knee Osteoarthritis: A three-Armed Randomized Trial. Ann Intern Med. 2006;145:12-20.

37] Vas J, Perea Milla E, Mendez C. Acupuncture and moxibustion as an adjunctive treatment for osteoarthritis of the knee - a large case series. Acup Med. 2004;221:23-8.

38] MacPherson H, Thomas K, Walters S, Fittler M. The York acupuncture safety study: prospective survey of 34,000 treatments by traditional acupuncturists. BMJ. 2001;323:486-7.

39] Kamoun N, Dziri C, Ben Salah FZ. Physiotherapy-Mesotherapy in the treatment of common cervicalgia. Rachis. 1998;10:47-150.

40] Palermo S, Riello R, Cammardella MP. TENS+ mesotherapy association in the therapy of cervico-brachialgia: preliminary data. Minerva Anesthesiologica. 1991;57:1084-85.

41] Piantoni D, Cotichelli E, Di Gianvito P. Clinical results of the multicentric experimentation. Giornale di Mesoterapia. 1981;1:60-3.

42] Ruggeri F, Bartoletti CA, Maggiori S. Clinical results of the multicentric experimentation. Giornale di Mesoterapia. 1981;1:47-9.

43] Mammucari M, Gatti M, Maggiori S, Sabato AF. Role of Mesotherapy in Musculoskeletal Pain: Opinions from the Italian Society of Mesotherapy. EvidenceBased Complementary and Alternative Medicine. 2012;2012:12.

44] Parrini M, Bergamaschi R, Azzoni R. Controlled study of acetylsalicylic acid efficacy by mesotherapy in lumbo-sciatic pain. Minerva Ortopedica Traumatologica. 2002;53(3):181-4.

45] Monticone M, Barbarino A, Testi C, Arzano S, Moschi A, Negrini S. Symptomatic efficacy of stabilizing treatment versus laser therapy for sub-acute low back pain with positive tests for sacroiliac dysfunction: a randomised clinical controlled trial with 1 year follow-up. Europa Medicophysica. 2004:40(4):263-8.

46] Costantino C, Marangio E, Coruzzi G. Mesotherapy versus systemic therapy in the treatment of acute low back pain: a randomized trial. Evidence-Based Complementary and Alternative Medicine. 2011;2011:6.

47] Di Cesare A, Giombini A, Di Cesare M, Ripani M, Vulpiani MC, Saraceni VM. Comparison between the effects of trigger point mesotherapy versus acupuncture points mesotherapy in the treatment of chronic low back pain: a short term randomized controlled trial. Complementary Therapies in Medicine. 2011;19(1):19- 26.

48] Narvarte DA, Rosset-Llobet J. Safety of subcutaneous microinjections (mesotherapy) in musicians. Medical Problems of Performing Artists. 2011;26(2):79- 83.

49] Carbonne A, Brossier F, Arnaud I. Outbreak of non tuberculous mycobacterial subcutaneous infections related to multiple mesotherapy injections. Journal of Clinical Microbiology. 2009;47(6):1961-4.

50] Meyruey M, Noaille-Degorce P, MerlierC, Chanez IP, Bousquet J. La mesotherapie, source de risques nouveaux. Rev Fr Allergol. 1986;26(1):27-8.

51] Herreros FOC, Moraes AM, Velho PENF. Mesotherapy: a bibliographical review. Ann Bras Dermatol. 2011;86(1):96-101.

52] Simons DG, Travell JG. Travell and Simons myofascial pain and dysfunction. The trigger point manual. Williams and Wilkins; 1999.

53] Lucas M, Macaskill P, Irwig L, Moran R, Bogduk N. Reliability of physical examination for diagnosis of myofascial trigger points: a systematic review of the literature. Clin J Pain. 2009;25:80-9.

54] Roland M, Fairbank JCT. The Roland-Morris disability questionnaire and the Oswestry disability questionnaire. Spine. 2000;31:15-24.

55] Fairbank JCT, Couper J, Davies JB, O'Brien J. The Oswestry low back pain disability questionnaire. Physiotherapy. 1980;66:271-3.

Appendix 1: Data collection form

Numéro Fiche : ☐☐   Nom : .... , Prénom : ....

Numéro de dossier : ☐☐☐☐   Numéro de téléphone : ☐☐ ☐☐☐ ☐☐☐

Acupuncture ☐   **Mésothérapie** ☐

Age : ☐☐ ans   Sexe : F ☐   M ☐

Profession : - Travail manuel ☐   - Sans profession ☐

 - Travail administratif ☐   - Retraité ☐

Ancienneté des douleurs : ....

Irradiation au MS : Oui ☐   Non ☐   Territoire : .C ☐

Signes associés:

- Fourmillement des mains :   oui ☐   non ☐
- Céphalée :   oui ☐   non ☐
- Vertige :   oui ☐   non ☐
- Acouphène :   oui ☐   non ☐

Traitement médicamenteux : .AA ☐   AINS ☐   Myorelaxants ☐   Aucun ☐

Rééducation : Oui ☐   Non ☐

Evolution :

	Evaluation initiale	Après A3 ou M1	Après A6 ou M2	Après A10 ou M3 (fin du TTT)
EVA				
Distance menton-sternum au repos				
Distance menton-sternum à la F				
Distance menton-sternum à l' E				
Distance menton-acromion RDte				
Distance menton-acromion RG				
Distance Tragus-acromion ILDte				
Distance Tragus-acromion ILG				
Distance C3- mur				
Distance C7- mur				

Appendix 2: Example of acupuncture points used

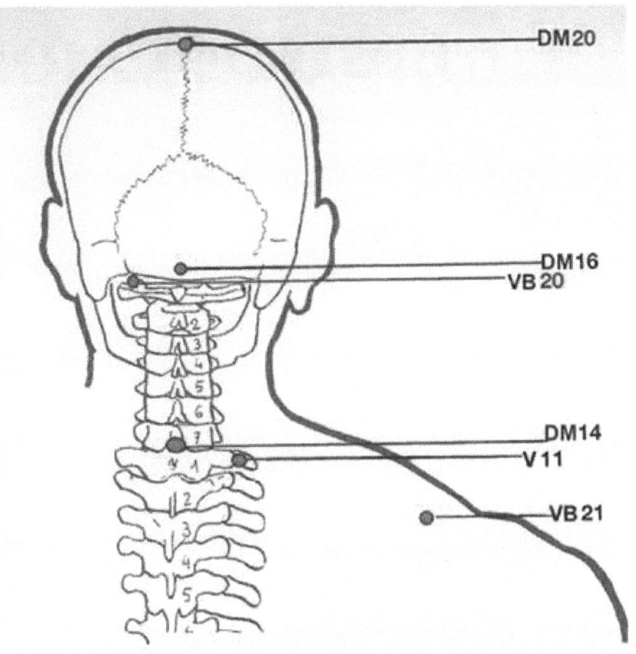